CU00409147

Take Your Life Back

The Real Cause of Migraines and How to Cure Them

Dawn Gregory

Table of Contents

Introduction

Migraines steal your life one day at a time. We suffer, learn to recognize our triggers, do what we can to cope. We live in fear of the next day lost to migraine.

We may depend on doctors who charge thousands of dollars for mediocre diagnoses and ineffective medications. We may get sympathy from our family and friends, who can see how much pain we're in but don't understand it. We commiserate with other migraineurs and come to believe there is no real solution. It seems there is no-one who can show us the way to a cure.

I am going to tell you why you get migraines and how you can cure them. It will not take thousands of dollars or drastic changes to your lifestyle. I am going to show you a simple and effective way to take your life back from migraines.

I am a migraineur, just like you, and I have managed to cure my own migraines.

I had my first migraine in December 1996, during my twelfth week of pregnancy. It was preceded by weeks of nausea, exhaustion, caffeine and nicotine withdrawal, and poor diet. I was living on protein shakes and prenatal vitamins, unable to prepare regular meals or eat them. Two weeks later, I lost the baby.

From that point, the migraines became progressively worse and more frequent. By 2005, I was losing two full days each week to the devastating pain. I tried career change, better nutrition, massage, meditation, and medication, and I quit drinking and did yoga. I found that, by doing those things, I could avoid migraines sometimes but not always. Some new factor would always creep into my life, and the migraines would take over again.

My training and experience are in computer databases. I specialize in collecting, organizing, and analyzing vast amounts of data. I have spent the better part of two decades collecting information about migraines and analyzing the patterns in the current treatment protocols. I have looked for gaps in the information and filled in the blanks. I experiment with the recommended treatments and keep track of what works for me and why.

I have returned to the research time and again, only to find one disempowering statement: No one knows why migraines occur.

I am here to tell you, that statement is wrong. I know why migraines occur. You probably do, too, but haven't been successful in using that knowledge to cure your migraines.

Migraines are caused by a toxic lifestyle that creates a buildup of toxins inside our bodies. Migraine triggers are the things we do or experience that create toxic conditions. Migraine treatments are designed to manage the pain and avoid subsequent attacks, but they don't address the root cause of built up toxins.

The cure for migraines is to fix the systems inside your body that are designed to process toxins. Once these systems are working correctly, exposure to toxic conditions will no longer cause migraines.

I am going to show you how you can cure your migraines. I'm not just talking about prevention or treatment, but an actual cure. You can use the information I am going to share, so you will never have to suffer from migraines again.

This past weekend I traveled halfway across the country and spent three days exposing myself to my entire range of migraine triggers. I stayed up until daylight three nights in a row. I slept a total of eight hours in three days. I pushed my limits of physical endurance throughout. I didn't eat well or drink nearly enough water. I drank alcohol. I exposed myself to a toxic urban environment and rode uncomfortable, jarring public transportation.

In the past, any one of these factors, for even one day, would have caused a severe migraine. Today, I came home exhausted but energized. Today, I have overcome all of these triggers and did not suffer a migraine.

I am going to show you how to cure your migraines, too. You can be free to live your life without the fear of losing another day to migraines. You can do the things you want to do, even if they have triggered migraines in the past. You can push your limits and come away unscathed.

You can take your life back from migraines.

Read this book to learn why you get migraines and how to cure them. You have nothing to lose and so many productive days to gain. Don't wait until the next migraine before you get started. Use the simple treatments I am going to show you, and you will never have to suffer from migraines again.

The Real Cause of Migraines

Migraines are caused by a toxic lifestyle. We repeatedly engage in behavior that exposes our bodies to toxins. This is not entirely our fault—the world we live in is highly toxic. Over time, toxins accumulate and get distributed all over the body.

If you continue ignoring the signs that you are poisoning yourself, a migraine is a very effective way for your body to get the attention it needs. A migraine is your body's way of screaming "stop!" in no uncertain terms.

Some people can live a toxic lifestyle constantly and never experience the pain of a migraine. Others go to great lengths to avoid toxic exposure and end up with chronic migraines anyway. Since you are still reading, I suspect you are on this end of the scale. So why do some people get migraines and others don't?

It is really a simple matter of the body's ability to manage toxic exposure. If your body can't process the toxins effectively, migraines are likely—and the alternatives are worse: cancer, diabetes, heart disease, death. Be grateful that you have migraines because they are preventing you from doing real harm to yourself.

Yes, I said that you should be grateful you have migraines. Of course, you will be even more grateful to not have them. Don't worry; we'll get there.

Migraine Triggers

Migraine triggers do not cause migraines. Migraine triggers expose your body to toxins. Accumulated toxins that your body can't eliminate are what cause a migraine.

To date, the most reliable method for managing migraines is to carefully document your migraines in a migraine journal. With sufficient data to analyze, you can identify your specific triggers and then modify your lifestyle to avoid them.

To create a migraine journal, you start with the date, time, and severity of a migraine, and the symptoms you are experiencing. Whenever the migraine gets better or worse, record the change and whatever you did in between. Once the migraine is finally over, add information about the possible triggers including foods you ate and what you did over the two days before the migraine started.

There are some great, easy-to-use tools for tracking your symptoms, frequency, severity, triggers, and treatments. This is very helpful in giving you the "big picture" of your migraines. If you've never kept a migraine journal before, you may want to try the Migraine Buddy app for your phone or the online journal at The Migraine Trust (http://www.migrainetrust.org/). If you want to keep it simple, buy a notebook and use it to track your migraines as I just described.

I used this method for many years and had some success at preventing migraines. Unfortunately, as you probably know, this approach is only preventative. It has several glaring flaws:

1. It is not always possible to avoid your triggers. Your job, your home, or the things you love to do may require that you expose yourself to your triggers.
2. Successfully avoiding all your known triggers will not prevent migraines. After some time, new triggers will pop up and send you back into a cycle of analysis, identification, and lifestyle changes.
3. Avoiding your triggers reduces the amount of toxins introduced into your body. It does not improve your body's ability to manage toxins.

With this method, migraines run your life. Wouldn't it be better if you could control your migraines instead of letting them control you?

In case you aren't convinced that migraine triggers fill your body with toxins, I am going to spend the rest of this chapter reviewing the most common migraine triggers, the toxins they create, and common strategies for dealing with them.

Stress

Stress, in its various forms, is the most common migraine trigger. This may include workplace stress, worry, fear, arguing, anger, crying, depression, anxiety, and even lack of sleep. Major life changes and chronic pain are stressful. The pain, fear, and depression resulting from chronic migraines will trigger more migraines.

Stress is an emotional response to the circumstances of our lives and can be extremely challenging to overcome. Unchecked, stress creates a cycle of ever-increasing stress.

Stress, in all its forms, creates a toxin called Adrenaline. While Adrenaline evolved to give us enhanced performance when survival is at stake, long-term exposure to Adrenaline is toxic. We cannot persist in a constant state of Adrenaline-charged, reactive behavior. Adrenaline is meant to give us a momentary boost of strength, reaction time, and clarity of thought. It is not meant to be a way of life.

Even though our odds of survival in the modern world are better than ever before, we live in a constant state of stress. Meditation, yoga, massage, and other relaxation techniques can help us overcome long-term stress, if applied consistently. They are helpful techniques for managing stress-related migraines.

Environmental Toxins

Exposure to toxins in the world around us is another very common migraine trigger. Toxins are absorbed into the body through our skin, eyes, and lungs. Environmental toxins include chemical cleaners and chemicals involved in manufacturing certain products. Allergens, such as tree and plant pollens, dust, and pet dander, are environmental toxins for some people. Pollution, carbon monoxide, and chlorine gas may be inhaled into the lungs unintentionally. Many beauty products, including makeup, skin cleansers, and moisturizer, contain chemicals that are absorbed through the skin and accumulated to toxic levels.

Environmental toxins are the hardest to overcome in preventing migraines. You aren't going to put on a gas mask every time you go outdoors. Getting away from environmental toxins may require that you move, change jobs, switch to new cleaning and beauty products, or get rid of your pets. These are all big changes, which are hard to make and have limited impact on preventing migraines. No matter where you go, there are going to be environmental toxins that will eventually trigger migraines.

Internal Chemistry

A whole range of triggers are related to our internal body chemistry, which we have limited ability to control. This includes monthly hormone cycles, prescribed medications, gum disease, injury, growth, illness, dehydration, and malnutrition.

These triggers change the body's internal chemical environment. Toxins may be introduced directly, through taking medication or being exposed to a pathogen that causes illness. Sometimes they are simply toxic by-products of the body's natural processes.

Some internal chemistry triggers are easily avoided. Prevent gum disease by flossing daily. Prevent dehydration by drinking more water. Prevent malnutrition by eating a balanced diet and using vitamin supplements. Other internal chemistry triggers cannot be avoided at all, and migraines seem inevitable.

Micro-Strain

A whole range of migraine triggers revolves around repeated, minute, corrective movements. These include excessive computer use or reading, reading with poor lighting or incorrect prescription lenses, wearing tight clothing or uncomfortable shoes, sleeping on an old mattress or a waterbed, shivering, TMJ or grinding your teeth, and any activity performed for long periods of time without concern for a healthy, ergonomically-sound body position.

Micro-strain is caused by incomplete movement of the small muscles required for precise motor control. Movement involves the release of chemicals that cause a muscle to contract. Normally, the muscle relaxes once it is fully contracted, and byproducts of the chemical reaction get carried away in the bloodstream.

With the types of activities that cause micro-strain, the muscles never get a chance to relax. When muscles do not relax after contracting, the chemical byproducts of normal movement stay "stuck" in the muscle tissues. This is why your muscles get sore during strength training exercises: Repeated contraction of the muscle, without allowing it to fully relax, causes a buildup of toxins which make the muscle sore later.

In the case of micro-strain, four factors combine to create a toxic condition through this normal body process:

1. The muscles involved are very small, so the entire tissue becomes saturated with toxic byproducts very quickly.
2. The activity causing the micro-strain tends to persist for hours instead of minutes, building up toxins throughout.

3. It becomes more difficult to finally relax the muscle and release the toxins after prolonged use.
4. All this is made worse by our tendency to repeat these activities day after day.

The solutions to micro-strain are very straightforward: Get new glasses; use better lighting; replace your mattress; wear comfortable clothes and shoes; see a specialist about your TMJ or grinding; and create an ergonomic workspace. Stretching, massage, and exercise can help. See a Chiropractor or Acupuncturist to improve your alignment and release pent-up tension.

Food Triggers

A long list of specific foods may trigger migraines in some people. I will discuss food triggers in more detail in later chapters. To briefly summarize, the foods tend to fall into these major groups:

- Highly processed foods, such as pork products, deli meats, and canned goods
- Fermented or cultured foods such as yogurt, sour cream, pickles, sauerkraut, cheese, alcohol, soy sauce
- Chemical food additives such as MSG, Saccharine, Aspartame
- Sweet foods including candy, pastry, and fruit
- Nutrient-dense foods like Brewer's yeast and liver

- Caffeine in coffee, tea, cola, chocolate, etc.
- Seeds of plants, including grains, beans, nuts, pods, and seeds

When specific foods trigger a migraine, something in the food is toxic for the body. It may be something obvious, such as the chemicals added to the food or the nutrients it contains. In other cases, the toxic effects of certain foods are not so obvious. They will become apparent as I tell you more about the cure for migraines.

How to Cure Migraines

A migraine is the body's way of putting a stop to all the abuse of a toxic modern lifestyle. When we persist in behaviors that are toxic, the poisons build up in our body. At some point, the body can't take any more and forces us to stop through the intense pain, confusion, and hypersensitivity known as a migraine.

We learn to avoid toxic behaviors and medicate the pain away, which poisons us even further. The migraines keep coming.

For most migraineurs, the problem is that our bodies are so filled with toxins that a day or two of reparation is not enough. We treat ourselves well until the toxins drop to a manageable level, and then we go back to our lives. The symptoms go away, but the underlying cause is still circulating inside us.

In holistic medicine, this condition is well-known and has a name: "bad blood." Bad blood doesn't refer to excess blood sugar, high cholesterol, or a feud with someone. Bad blood is toxic, for sure, but it won't necessarily kill you (yet).

Good blood brings nourishment to your body tissues in the form of energy and oxygen. After making its delivery, the blood picks up the byproducts of metabolism and carries them back to the liver to be filtered, processed, and discarded. Bad blood is so filled with toxins that it drops off a dose of poison at every stop and doesn't have any capacity to pick up more. The tissues fill up with toxins that are overflowing in the bloodstream.

To cure migraines, you need to clean up your blood. The key to making this happen is getting your liver to do its job effectively.

The liver is the chemical intelligence in your body. It is not just a passive filter; it is literally your CPU: Chemical Processing Unit. The liver takes in both the "fresh" chemicals from the food we eat and the "rotten" chemicals returned by the circulatory system. Its job is to analyze all these chemicals and decide what to do with them.

When the liver is working well, it converts carbohydrates to energy and sends them out into the bloodstream. It captures fats and stores them for later use. It breaks down proteins into their parts (amino acids) and sends them where they are needed. It stores and distributes vitamins and minerals. And it captures toxins returned from the tissues and breaks them down so they can be discarded. The liver has an awful lot to do.

Of course, this is just a general overview, but it explains the complexity of the liver's job. For the purposes of curing migraines, the liver needs to perform optimally to clean the bad blood. If the liver is deficient, blood toxins accumulate, and over time, with new triggers, a migraine will occur.

I'm a math geek, so it made sense to write some equations:

Deficient Liver + Toxins + Time = Bad Blood

Bad Blood + Trigger = Migraine

This is purely descriptive. You aren't going to be able to "solve" the equation to cure migraines. The liver is the key to solving this equation because it can be healed:

Healthy Liver + Toxins + Time = Good Blood

Good Blood + Trigger = No Migraine

A healthy liver cancels the effects of bad blood, and then no amount of toxins, triggers, and time will cause a migraine.

The key to curing migraines is to get your liver back to full operation. You can't do this by taking medications. Medications are unknown chemicals the liver doesn't recognize, and stress the liver even further. However, there is a powerful, freely available medicine that can heal your liver in just a few weeks. It is probably growing right outside your door.

The Miracle Migraine Cure

Do you ever gaze out at your beautifully manicured, chemically-treated lawn and curse those little yellow heads that just keep popping up everywhere in spite of your best efforts? Please stop doing that. Those smiling yellow faces aren't there to taunt you; they are there because you need them.

Dandelion is traditionally known as a "blood cleanser" and "liver tonic." Dandelions show up in the spring when our circulatory system is clogged with toxins from a sedentary and poorly-nourished winter season. They show up just when we need them, shining brightly to remind us so. In earlier times, people integrated Dandelion greens into their springtime menu because they were plentiful and available before most other edibles. They also ate Dandelion to recharge their systems for the season of hard work to come.

In modern times, our winter diet is nutritionally sound. We have such a variety of foods available that we don't miss out on vital nutrients just because of the season. Instead, we have a toxic environment that stresses our bodies and creates disease. We have toxic foods that are impregnated with chemicals and genetically-engineered for maximum productivity, with minimum concern about their health effects. We have cancer, heart disease, diabetes, and, of course, migraines. And the Dandelions keep showing up everywhere because we need them more than ever. Please stop cursing them. Eat them!

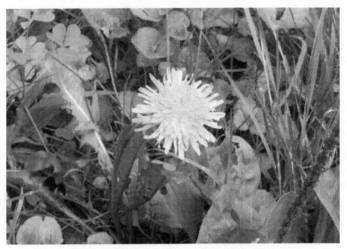

Dandelion is a migraine miracle

When I first started writing this book, I woke up with a migraine one morning (maybe writing about migraines is a migraine trigger). I took ¼ of a teaspoon of magical Dandelion Root tincture right away. After an hour, the pain was gone, but the tension and grogginess were still there. I took another ¼ teaspoon and, an hour after that, the migraine was totally gone.

Dandelion is high in vitamins A and C as well as iron, potassium, and choline. It is specifically targeted to liver cleansing, improves digestion, and is a natural diuretic and a mood stabilizer. Dandelion may have interactions with medications. If you are taking a prescription medicine, or if you are pregnant or nursing, be smart and consult your doctor before trying it.

Dandelion leaf is a diuretic. Do not take it with diuretic medications. Drink plenty of water while you are using it, or you will get dehydrated, and that will give you a migraine.

Here are three ways you can use Dandelion:

1. Go outside and pick some fresh Dandelion leaves and flowers (not from a chemically-treated lawn). Discard the stems. Saute the leaves and flowers in butter with a little garlic. Yum!
2. Make an infusion by putting the leaves and flowers (no stems) and/or the root into one cup of water. Heat the water almost to boiling; then turn off the heat, cover the pan, and let it sit for twenty minutes. Strain out the plant parts and drink the liquid.
3. If it is winter or you live in the city and there are no fresh Dandelions available, you can purchase a tincture of Dandelion from a reputable herbalist or even on Amazon.com.

Now that you know what to do and how to do it, I won't be offended if you put the book down and go outside to pick some flowers. The rest can wait until you get back.

To heal your liver and clean the toxins from your blood, the following "prescription" can be used.

Dandelion Protocol:

1. Take Dandelion three times a day for one week, either sautéed leaves and flowers, one cup of infusion, or 1 mL tincture. Drink a large glass of water with each dose to offset the diuretic effects.
2. Reduce to one time per day for one week.
3. Reduce to every other day for two weeks.
4. Take as needed when you are exposed to migraine triggers or if you start experiencing symptoms.

You can continue to take Dandelion on a daily basis if you are frequently exposing yourself to migraine triggers. Please remember to drink at least 8-12 ounces of water with each dose to avoid dehydration. After three to four weeks, you should reduce the frequency and see if you can get to the point where it is only needed on occasion.

More Intensive Treatment

If you are still getting migraines after the second week, or if you finish the four-week sequence and still get migraines regularly, there is another, more potent herb for liver cleansing. This one is also likely to be growing right outside your door.

Proceed with caution! This is potent medicine, a powerful diuretic, may cause diarrhea, and has drug interactions!

Yellow Dock, *Rumex Crispus*, is an even more invasive, less welcomed weed that is a powerful herbal remedy for toning the liver. Not only prolific, this weed grows into a giant: three to four feet tall if left unchecked. Toward the end of summer, it produces foot-long spears containing thousands of rust-colored seeds. This plant is anything but beautiful, and like the Dandelion, it spreads quickly, so we put a lot of effort into eradicating it from our yards.

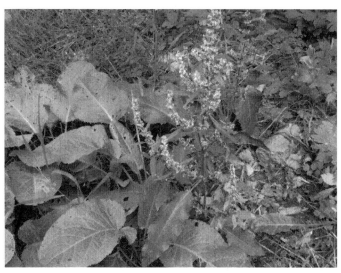

Yellow Dock is for deep cleansing

There are several varieties of Dock and they are all highly medicinal. Yellow Dock is specific for liver cleansing. It is also very high in iron, so if you tend to be anemic or have "low blood sugar," it is a good choice. It improves digestion and helps treat eczema, psoriasis, arthritis, and yeast infections. It is a potent laxative, so it should be taken in moderation.

Yellow Dock is truly a wonderful, all-purpose remedy, growing right outside the door. The leaves can be used, but the most potent medicine is in the roots, which are thick, deep, and yellow in color. Dig up the roots of first year plants (the ones without seeds) during the fall harvest season. Clean them and split lengthwise into long strips, or slice across the root to make small discs.

The fresh or dried roots can be used to make an infusion using the method I described above: Add the roots to 1 cup water; heat until almost boiling; remove from heat, cover, and allow it to sit for twenty minutes.

You can purchase Yellow Dock online as a dried, powdered root or in a tincture. For intense cleansing, the powdered root is preferable. For a gradual effect, you may want to try the tincture in limited doses.

Yellow Dock may cause severe interactions with some medications, such as diuretics and blood thinners.

I have used Yellow Dock for intense liver cleansing and have to give it the credit for finally curing my migraines. Dandelion is fairly gentle and works well as a preventative measure. Dock is truly deep-cleansing. It is not to be used carelessly.

Intense Cleansing Protocol:

1. Prepare one cup of root infusion using fresh or powdered root. Drink one-half of a cup ONLY, and refrigerate the rest.
2. Stay near a bathroom and drink LOTS of extra water. Extreme diarrhea may occur with high doses.
3. Drink the remaining one-half cup of infusion the next morning.
4. Avoid fruits, yogurt, and any other foods that will cause loose stool.
5. If you get a headache, drink more water.

After two to three days, your body will return to normal, and you should feel better all over. You may have even lost some weight. This protocol can be repeated after a month or so if your migraines return. You can also try very small doses of 1-3 drops. However, it should not be used on a regular basis. This is only for intensive deep cleansing.

Further Treatment

Returning your liver to normal function will give you resistance to migraine triggers. Use Dandelion any time you are exposed to your triggers, or if you feel a migraine coming on. If you continue to get migraines, it is time to consider additional factors.

It is a good idea to enlist the help of a holistic practitioner such as a certified herbalist. You can visit the American Herbalists Guild website (http://www.americanherbalistsguild.com) for a list of resources in your area. Tell your doctor you want to integrate a holistic practitioner into your treatment plan. If he or she disagrees, fire him or her and get a new doctor who understands the benefit of a holistic approach.

Your internal organs form a complex network that makes your body function. If your liver is back to normal but you are still having migraines, you can look to the function of other organs and repair them, too. A holistic practitioner will be able to make the best diagnosis, considering all of your symptoms, and prescribe the most effective treatment.

I am going to review the organs that have specific roles in eliminating toxins from your body. The function of each organ is related to specific migraine symptoms and triggers. If you still have migraines after healing your liver, look to these other organs.

Organ	Symptoms	Food Triggers
Gall Bladder	Right-side headache over eye	Fatty foods, chemicals in food
Kidney	Back of head, noise / jolt sensitive, joints ache	Dehydration, protein-rich foods
Small Intestine	Allergies, rash, sinus headache	Beans, grains, nuts, seeds
Large Intestine	Nausea, IBS	Cheese, fermented foods, caffeine
Lymphatics	Neck and shoulder ache	Sweet foods
Skin	Hot/cold, sensitive to touch	Salty foods
Lung	Anxiety, exhaustion	Smoking, dehydration

Incidentally, the liver is associated with light sensitivity, left-side headache, nausea, vomiting, and consuming alcohol or too much of **any** kind of food. Once the liver is restored, the remaining symptoms and triggers are more clearly associated with specific organs.

I am going to give you an overview of the relationship between these waste processing organs and migraines. A trained practitioner will be able to give you a more detailed diagnosis.

Gallbladder

The gallbladder is a small, pouch-like organ connected to the liver. It is basically a storage area for the liver. It helps the liver with both fat digestion and eliminating unidentified chemicals.

The liver generates bile, which is used to digest fats. Any excess bile that is created will be sent to the gallbladder for storage until it is needed. Excess fat in the diet makes the liver create more bile, so the gallbladder has to work harder. It is just a little sac; it isn't meant to work so hard.

The liver also uses the gallbladder for temporary storage of chemicals it doesn't recognize. Specifically, synthetic chemicals, which have no place in the body, are sent to the gallbladder along with bile. These include artificial sweeteners, chemicals used in packaging and canning, any poisons you decide to consume, and environmental toxins absorbed into the bloodstream. The chemicals get returned along with the bile when the liver is processing fat. Since the liver doesn't know what to do with these chemicals, it wraps them in fat and sends them to be stored away safely in fatty deposits throughout the body.

Gallbladder deficiency is associated with oily skin, dandruff, twitching, and migraines on the right side of the head. You may also experience bloating after meals, especially if they are high in fat.

The gallbladder is closely tied to the liver, and herbal remedies for the liver work for the gallbladder, too. Dandelion is the best herbal remedy for the gallbladder. By using it to treat your liver, you should be well on your way to healing the gallbladder already.

More importantly, fat consumption must be carefully controlled. It isn't just the quantity of fat you are eating, but the quality. Fat is very volatile and easily turns toxic with light, heat, and time.

Since the 1980s, we've been taught that fat is bad. Not only does fat make you fat, it causes a whole host of diseases. Recently, scientists have begun to understand that not all fat is bad. Your body needs fat. Your brain, especially, needs fat. The latest research demonstrates that some fats are very good for you. There are also some fats that are very, very bad for you.

All plant-based fats in their whole, natural form are good for you, including avocado and nuts. When fats are extracted from plants, they become less healthy. The harder it is to extract the oils, the less healthy the resulting product is. For the most part, vegetable-based oils are toxic. The processes needed to extract the oils will damage the fat molecules, and the oil contains toxins right off the shelf. Removing oils from animal fat, fruits, and seeds is much easier and produces oils that are good for you.

The best fats you can eat are:

1. Ghee (clarified butter)
2. Palm or Palm kernel oil
3. Almond, Olive, or Coconut oil
4. Sesame oil
5. Butter
6. Pure Lard (make sure it has no hydrogenated or partially hydrogenated oils added)

Basically, no other oils should be used in your diet, ever. Cooking temperature, exposure to air and light, and aging of the oils create toxins and make them unhealthy. Just like the diminutive Dandelion, fats need to be appreciated more and treated well.

Kidneys

The kidneys control the flow of liquid in the body and filter the byproducts of protein metabolism (Urea) from the blood. The kidneys control the concentration of electrolytes in the body and discard any excess in the urine. Dehydration has a severe effect on the kidneys, as does a diet high in protein.

Dehydration is becoming widely recognized as an underlying factor in many chronic disease patterns, including migraines. Most recommendations for migraine treatment already mention increased water intake and supplementing with essential electrolytes, such as

Potassium and Magnesium. Your kidneys need sufficient water and electrolytes to maintain chemical equilibrium in the body.

If you are extremely sensitive to noise or jolts during or between migraines, the kidneys should be considered. Kidneys are associated with headaches behind the ears, in the back of the head. Aches and pains in the joints are also an indicator of low kidney function.

The first step to healing the kidneys is staying properly hydrated. Drinking room temperature water helps the kidneys return to normal function. Cranberries and (real) cranberry juice have been found to improve kidney function. Dandelion will also help restore kidney function.

When you eat excessive amounts of protein, the kidneys have to work harder. If your urine is cloudy, excess protein is effecting your kidney function. Protein should be approximately 30 percent of your daily calorie intake, fifty to sixty grams per day on average. You need more only if you are pregnant or bodybuilding. Protein supplements may be to blame for low kidney function. Try to distribute your protein intake throughout the day, consuming fifteen to twenty grams, three times a day.

Proper electrolyte balance is also essential for kidney function. Electrolytes include Sodium, Potassium, Calcium, Magnesium, and even Chlorine. Electrolytes are nutrients that carry an electrical charge, either positive or negative. The electrical charge makes electrolytes chemically reactive with other elements they encounter inside the body.

The kidneys control the levels of electrolytes in the bloodstream; if the levels are too low, the kidneys restore electrolyte balance by eliminating water. When electrolyte levels are too high, kidney damage can occur. Drink more water!

Small Intestine

The small intestine is where the important parts of our digestive process take place. Food is broken down with digestive juices, and nutrients are absorbed through the walls of the intestine. When the small intestine is fully functioning, we get the most benefit from the food we eat, and everything moves through in twelve to twenty-four hours.

When the small intestine is not working properly, you will get gas and bloating, congestion and inflammation, acne, rashes, allergies, and sinus headaches. A surprising amount of the immune system is based in the small Intestine. If you get sick frequently, the small intestine may be damaged.

If your migraines are triggered by allergies, weather and altitude changes, grains, beans, or nuts, the small intestine may be playing a role. This is even more likely if you are gluten intolerant or have frequent bouts of diarrhea.

To heal the small intestine, you first want to stop eating any foods that are the seeds of plants, i.e., seeds, nuts, beans, peas, pods, peanuts, and **all cereal grains**. Gluten is well-known as a cause of damage to the small intestine, so a gluten-free diet is a good start.

All plant seeds contain *Anti Nutrient Factors* (ANFs), chemicals that actually prevent the digestion of nutrients. *Phytate* steals minerals such as Sodium, Calcium, Magnesium, Iron, and Zinc from your body. *Protease inhibitors* block protein-digesting enzymes. *Lectins* cause gut inflammation and autoimmune disease. *Polyphenols* steal Iron and Zinc and inhibit digestive secretions. ANFs evolved in seeds so they wouldn't be digested when consumed, and they could survive to sprout another day.

Zinc deficiency is associated with loss of small intestine function. Damage to the intestine reduces its ability to absorb Zinc from food. Supplementing with Zinc is essential to staying healthy when the small intestine is damaged.

Herbal remedies for the small intestine include Slippery Elm, Yarrow, and Echinacea. Slippery Elm is a powder extracted from the inner bark of the tree. Dissolved in cold water and then heated, it forms a gel-like substance similar to Metamucil. Slippery Elm is cooling and soothing to the small intestine and will help improve your digestion.

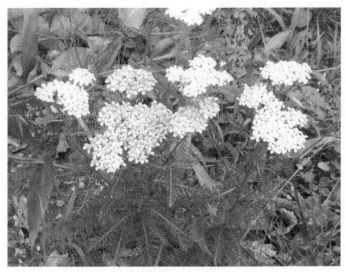

Yarrow heals damaged tissue

Yarrow is a common wildflower found throughout North America and is easiest to use in tincture form. It is for repairing damaged tissue anywhere in the body. Fresh Yarrow tincture will help repair any porosity in the intestine, particularly if you are gluten intolerant. Incidentally, it is also great for cuts, scrapes, burns, and rashes, so get a big bottle and use it frequently!

Echinacea is anti-bacterial and will be helpful for any immunity concerns caused by damage to the intestine. If you have allergies, congestion, or inflammation, it will assist in relieving the symptoms while your intestine recovers.

Large Intestine

The large intestine is the pathway to eliminating solid waste. Yes, I'm talking about poop. If you are frequently constipated or alternate between diarrhea and constipation, your large intestine may not be working properly.

Constipation causes the buildup of toxins that should have been eliminated. Dehydration, stress, lack of fiber in the diet, and too much caffeine may be to blame. You know the drill: Drink more water; eat more fiber; poop well; and be healthy. Don't use laxatives! They may help you get moving, but they will damage your large intestine even further. Avoid cheese, dairy products, and processed meats. Try probiotics to improve your digestion.

Poor functioning of the large intestine may indicate a Magnesium deficiency, and low Magnesium levels are known to aggravate migraines. Magnesium is essential for building strong bones and teeth, maintaining heart rhythm, and regulating blood sugar levels. Low Magnesium contributes to a whole range of health problems including fibromyalgia, diabetes, cardiovascular disease, and migraine. Magnesium supplements have a laxative effect and are specifically indicated for large intestine deficiency.

Stress is a major factor in large intestine function. Meditate to calm the mind. Drink less coffee. Exercise more! Get your body moving to get your bowels moving. A nice long walk after dinner is a great remedy. Stay calm and sleep well.

Chamomile is the gentlest herbal remedy for the large intestine. It helps you relax and helps you sleep. Have a nice cup of Chamomile tea before bed and start moving again in the morning.

Lymphatics

The lymphatic system is a secondary waste removal system for your cells (blood being the primary). You've heard of lymph nodes, those little glands in your neck, armpits, and chest that get swollen when you're sick. Lymph is cellular waste that accumulates in body tissues, outside the blood vessels. Lymph nodes are miniature filters that remove waste products from lymph as it flows through lymphatic channels. The tonsils, adenoids, thymus, and spleen are part of the lymphatic system.

The lymphatic system plays a critical role in immunity and toxin elimination. If the lymphatic system is working properly, lymph drains into the lymphatic channels, filters through the lymph nodes, and gets discarded back into the bloodstream just before it enters the heart.

When the lymphatic system is not working correctly, lymph gets stuck in the tissues and accumulates under the skin. The knots in your muscles after strenuous labor are pockets of accumulated lymph.

If you are subject to migraines due to micro-strain, as I am, your body is not disposing of lymph effectively. You may get frequent neck and shoulder aches. The tension and the toxins will build up from repeated activities that cause strain, and lead to a migraine.

Massage is a great way to release the accumulated lymph from your tissues and get it flowing again. Yoga postures that twist the body and Acupuncture or Chiropractic treatments may be helpful.

Herbal remedies include Echinacea, Calendula, and Red Clover. As I already mentioned, Echinacea is anti-bacterial; it supports your immune system and reduces the toxins stored in lymph. Calendula encourages circulation, not just in the bloodstream, but in the lymphatic system, too. Red Clover and Calendula are known as *Lymphagogue* herbs, which have the specific action of cleansing and restoring the lymphatic system.

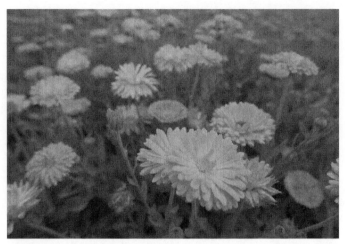

Calendula restores the flow (photo by Leonid Shcheglov)

Skin

The skin is the largest organ and plays a major role in removing waste from the body. Lymph that is not disposed through the lymphatic channels works its way to the skin's surface and is removed from the body along with the toxins it contains. The skin eliminates water and salts that accumulate in tissues near its surface.

If your skin is dry and rough, if you use lotions made with chemicals, or if you are highly sensitive to chemicals in your environment, the skin may be a concern. You may find that your migraines are triggered by very salty foods, especially those containing artificial salts such as MSG or nitrites.

A long, hot shower or bath will remove the toxins from your skin and give you a chance to rehydrate. Exfoliating with loofah, pumice, or salt removes dead skin, opens pores, and smooths the surface. Oiling yourself with natural oils, such as Almond, Coconut, or Palm Kernel oil, makes your skin supple and creates a stronger barrier to your environment. Oh yes, and drink more water!

Lungs

The lungs bring oxygen into the body where it is absorbed by the blood and carried off to the cells. When the blood returns, the lungs extract carbon dioxide and send it back to the world.

Lack of oxygen makes you tired. For the most part, we don't breathe deeply enough, and our bodies are deprived of vital oxygen. Carbon dioxide accumulates in unused areas of the lungs, and these areas cannot replenish the blood effectively. When you are stressed, nervous, arguing, or crying, your chest gets tight, and breathing is even less effective. Smoking and congestion may compound the problem further.

Breathe deeply! A full breath in takes five seconds or more, and nearly as long to let out. It fills your chest and expands your stomach. You should feel it all the way to your backbone. A handful of full, deep breaths will calm your mind, ease stress, and give you more energy. Give it a try now! We all need to breathe more deeply.

Aerobic exercises, a.k.a. cardio training, will help improve your lung capacity, so you will breathe deeper even at rest. Yoga is also helpful for the lungs. Yoga is not only about complicated postures or bending your body in unique ways; it is about the breath. Breathing and moving in harmony will bring you back to health.

Other Systems

The body is a complex machine, and I have limited the focus of this discussion to the organs that remove toxins from the body. In the multifaceted condition that is migraine, other systems play the role of triggers: They create toxins that can trigger migraine episodes.

The Endocrine system is responsible for hormones in the body. Hormones are basically chemical messages that inhibit or enhance body functions. The Endocrine system includes the thyroid and parathyroid; the adrenal, pituitary, and pineal glands; and the hypothalamus, pancreas, ovaries, and testes. The hormones released by the Endocrine system are part of the body's natural controls, but they can accumulate in the bloodstream and result in a toxic condition. For example, it is common for women to have migraines around their menstrual cycle, and this is thought to be a result of menstrual hormone production.

The Musculoskeletal system forms the structure of the body and provides the ability to move. We have seen that movement may cause migraines due to the overuse of muscles. Muscle imbalance, due to growth or injuries, can also cause migraines by placing undue strain on specific muscle groups.

The Nervous system is commonly considered a source of migraines. Inflammation in the vagus nerve, which connects to the base of the brain, has been associated with migraines in various studies. Medical researchers have found that stimulating the vagus nerve during a migraine episode will relieve migraine symptoms.

Clearly, migraine is a disease that has potential triggers coming from every area of the body. Fully restoring a healthy condition may require contributions from a variety of disciplines. Your doctor can review your symptoms and order tests to diagnose specific problems. A holistic practitioner will review your whole body and provide treatment to restore balance among these systems. Chiropractors, Acupuncturists, massage therapists, and other specialists should be consulted for specific concerns. It is essential to get multiple perspectives on your treatment plan to get the best possible outcome.

Migraine-Free Life

What a great concept, living without migraines. You now have the tools to make it a reality: Repair your liver, cleanse your blood, treat deficiencies in toxin management, and diagnose other concerns related to your specific triggers.

Now for the bad news; a migraine-free life **does require lifestyle changes**. Well, you already knew that, but the changes aren't necessarily what you think. You don't have to stop doing things that have triggered migraines in the past. Using the Dandelion protocol and other suggestions I've made, you don't have to give up the things you love.

What you do need to give up are the foods that are damaging your liver. One of these foods is the bad fats I told you about in the section on gall bladder. Here I am going to tell you about three more: alcohol, sugar, and chemically-processed food.

It is absolutely critical to your overall health and continuing to stay migraine-free that you reduce or eliminate these four things in your diet. If you slip up from time to time or give yourself a treat on occasion, it's OK. The important thing is to **stop consuming these things regularly**. Having french fries once in a while probably won't hurt; having them every day will.

Limit Alcohol

Migraine symptoms are almost identical to the symptoms of a hangover: confused thinking, exhaustion, sensitivity to light and sound, head and body aches, nausea and vomiting. Yet, with a hangover, we have no doubt as to what caused it. We know that pouring alcohol into our bodies can result in a hangover when done in excess. We do it anyway and pay for it the next day.

Alcohol puts a burden on your liver to process the excess carbohydrates it contains and to eliminate the toxic by-products of alcohol from your bloodstream. Excessive alcohol consumption results in Cirrhosis, physical damage to the liver. Interestingly, women are more likely to get Cirrhosis than men, just as women are more likely to get migraines than men. Cirrhosis shares symptoms with migraine, such as fatigue, confusion, and nausea.

If you have suffered from migraines for any period of time, you probably limit your alcohol intake already. If you get migraines and still drink alcohol regularly, you may need to consider whether it is worthwhile. Alcohol will definitely increase the occurrence of migraines.

Alcohol is one of several substances we consume far too often and become addicted to, and it has a devastating impact on our health and well-being. Alcohol provides no benefit to the body and causes weight gain, dehydration, and chronic health problems. Reducing or eliminating alcohol will help you stay migraine-free and will make your life better, too.

Eliminate Sugar

Recent studies have shown that sugar will stress and eventually cause damage to the liver. This is particularly true of fructose, the sugar found in fruit, and the high-fructose corn syrup that is found in so many packaged foods. You can find a lot of useful information about the negative health effects of sugar on the Sugar Science website (http://www.sugarscience.org).

The liver's primary responsibility is breaking down sugar, so it can be used as energy. When we eat too much sugar, the liver is overwhelmed by responsibility and stops working efficiently.

Here's the catch: We all eat too much sugar.

Sugar hides in foods we don't even perceive as being sweet, like pasta and tomato sauce. Sugar in the modern supermarket has over sixty different names and is hiding in nearly three-fourths of packaged foods! Never mind soda, candy, and desserts: Even foods we believe are "healthy" may be loaded with sugar, including yogurt, smoothies, granola bars, fruit juice, and "unsweetened" breakfast cereals.

The latest recommendation is a **maximum** of twenty-five grams of added sugar per day for women, thirty-eight grams per day for men. A single can of soda has a full day's worth of sugar!

Like alcohol, sugar added to the diet is completely useless from a nutritional perspective. Also, like alcohol, sugar is extremely addictive! If you don't believe it, just wait until you try to give it up. I personally had stronger and more irrational cravings when trying to give up sugar than I did when trying to give up alcohol. Giving up sugar may be the single most difficult thing I have ever done. And, like most difficult things, it was extremely rewarding. Not only did I lose weight, it was also my first step toward getting control over migraines.

Eliminating sugar is a key part of curing your migraines for good. Many people find the "cold turkey" method is the only way to do it. Throw away any packaged food that contains sugar; pour out your sodas and fruit juices; stop buying sweets; and say no to dessert. When ads for Dairy Queen or Little Debbie come on TV, walk out of the room and go have a glass of water.

Of course, this extreme approach may be impossible, especially if your family is addicted to sugar, too. For a more gradual approach, you may find the following strategies helpful:

Read the label: Learn to read ingredient labels, starting with the total grams of sugar per serving. With a maximum of twenty-five to thirty-eight grams allowed per day, you will soon find that most packaged foods have at least half your daily allotment. Also check the ingredients for high fructose corn syrup, and don't buy foods that contain it.

By learning to look at the total sugar in a food, you will find a few "gems" that don't add up to excessive sugar. Most dark chocolate, for example, is less than ten grams per serving.

Drink more water: In addition to helping you detox and improving your overall health, drinking water can kill your sugar cravings. Many of the cravings we experience for specific foods, especially sugar, are actually thirst. Drink more water all the time, and your sugar cravings will gradually go away.

Substitute fruit: When you really need something sweet, eat a piece of fruit. Dr. Joel Fuhrman has a great recipe for an ice cream substitute that is just mashed banana and cocoa powder, frozen. Don't worry too much about the fructose in fruit; the variety of nutrients and the fiber in fruit make up for it, as long as you eat fruit within reason. Fruit juice does not have these benefits. Dried fruit ALL has added sugar: It is not fruit; it is candy.

Shop the fringe: The outer sections of the supermarket tend to have whole, natural foods while the inner aisles are filled with packaged, processed, over-sweetened foods. Focus your shopping to the outer areas of the supermarket where foods don't need labels, and you're avoiding sugar automatically! Stay away from the bakery, though.

Learn about GI: Glycemic Index, or GI, is a measure of the body's ability to process the carbohydrates in food. The liver is responsible for processing carbs, so GI basically measures how much work the liver has to do to digest a food. A lower GI means the food is better for your liver. Sugar is at the top of the GI scale with a rating of 100. Lower GI foods (below 40) may have sugar in them, but don't have the same damaging effects on your liver. You can look up the Glycemic Index of almost any food on the University of Sydney's website: http://www.glycemicindex.com.

Avoid Chemicals Disguised as Food

The next time you're at the grocery store, pick up a pretty-colored box of breakfast cereal and examine the ingredients list. If you take out the sugar, over-processed grains, and unhealthy oils, what is left? A long list of synthetic vitamins added to make up for the nutrients lost during processing and a perhaps longer list of chemicals for flavoring, coloring, and preserving shelf life. Now, what is left? A sprinkling of raisins or almond slivers? This is not food!

So-called food manufacturers use the cheapest ingredients available and turn them into palatable products through the "miracle of modern chemistry." They dress up the products in pretty packages and promote them with irresistibly cute ads on TV. By the time the product makes it to your breakfast table, it bears no resemblance to food. Your kids may love it, but they shouldn't be eating it either.

Eating is for nourishing your body with the things it needs and avoiding things that cause it harm. Eating things that are chemically manipulated to look and taste good is unhealthy. Eating lots of things your body doesn't need leads to toxic levels of chemical by-products in your blood and a myriad of chronic diseases, including migraine.

Chemical toxins can accumulate in the body from almost any kind of food when it is prepared improperly or eaten in excess. This problem multiplies when we also consume a daily dose of chemicals along with our food. The liver has to work harder to figure out what to do with all these chemicals it does not understand.

Chemicals used for preserving and coloring foods have long been recognized as unhealthy. More recently, scientists have discovered that many other synthetic ingredients in food, including fillers and vitamins, may be just as concerning. Synthetic vitamins lack the companion chemicals that occur in natural foods and enhance their effectiveness. Fillers cause damage to our digestive system and create a toxic buildup of undigested food.

Modern chemistry is hiding in nearly every packaged food. It is also hiding in "whole, natural" foods that have been chemically or genetically modified to improve productivity, appearance, or disease and pest resistance. Specifically, a large percentage of soy, corn, and peanut crops in the US are genetically engineered. Beef and dairy products raised on corn contain these chemicals, too, along with the antibiotics and hormones they are fed so they will survive and grow quickly. Most produce contains chemical by-products of its production process.

A whole industry has grown up around foods that don't contain chemicals, which carry a premium price tag. The natural and organic food industries are generating billions in revenue by exploiting our fears about chemicals hiding in food. For migraineurs, those fears are very real. The benefit to your health is worth the additional cost.

For the purposes of migraine treatment, try starting with the big stuff, and work your way toward the purest food possible. First, make sure you aren't eating the artificial colors, flavors, and preservatives that have obvious detrimental effects. As you work to eliminate sugar and processed oils from your diet, you will find it easier to avoid fillers and artificial vitamins, too, as these tend to be found in the same foods.

Your taste for food will start to change. Preparing food yourself from whole, natural ingredients takes some practice, and, over time, you will find that processed foods just don't taste good anymore. At this point, you will start to notice the difference between an organic tomato and its chemically-produced counterpart. Grass-fed beef and organic dairy products taste like nature intended, and the factory-farmed versions don't even come close. Your taste buds and your body will thank you!

Drink More Water

Just in case you missed it, drink more water! This alone will not cure your migraines, but it is an essential piece of the puzzle.

Keep track of the water you are drinking to make sure you are meeting your daily minimum. The recommended minimum in ounces per day is half your body weight in pounds: If you weigh 150 pounds, you should drink seventy-five ounces of water each day. That is a minimum; it is better to drink more if you can.

If you are having trouble getting to your daily minimum, why not try a water-tracker app for your phone? They can remind you throughout the day to drink more water and keep a tally of exactly how much you need to reach your goal.

Coffee is not water; soda is not water; juice is not water; sports drinks are not water; even (chemically) flavored water is not water! Water is water. Learning to enjoy drinking water is one of the best things you can do for your body and for staying migraine-free for life.

Last and Very Important

The mouth is the most direct reflection of what is happening inside your body. If you are healthy, your mouth will be healthy, and your breath will smell good. Experienced holistic practitioners can actually look at your tongue and identify any deficiencies in your internal organs from the color, texture, and patterns they see. The eyes may be windows to the soul, but the mouth is the window into the body.

Good dental hygiene is critical to staying migraine-free. Poor dental hygiene leads to tooth decay and gum disease, which create excess bacteria in your mouth. The bacteria leaks into your stomach and sends toxins to your liver and small intestine. Gum disease has been linked to headaches, arthritis, respiratory disease, diabetes, heart disease, memory loss, and even some forms of cancer.

Consistent oral care is essential, including brushing, flossing, and regular visits to the dentist. For years, I've searched for a way to get better at the flossing habit, with little success. Recently, I learned of the concept of "micro-habits" and was able to turn this into consistent flossing every day. I encourage you to give it a try if the flossing habit is challenging for you, too.

A micro-habit is a (positive) action that takes almost no thought and less than fifteen seconds to perform. The idea behind micro-habits is there are no excuses. They are so simple and fast, you can even fit it in just before bed if you managed to put it off all day. When repeated consistently over time, micro-habits turn into full-blown, lifelong habits.

You can get started with the micro-habit, "floss one tooth every day." Flossing one tooth every day may seem silly, but it builds the habit. Once you get in the habit of doing it every single day, before long, you will find that you floss two teeth, then three, then four, and, in no time at all, you're actually flossing your whole mouth every day. Within two or three weeks, your mouth will be much heathier, and you will have reduced your risk for a whole host of nasty diseases, including migraines.

Migraine Science

It may seem strange to read a whole book about migraines without any discussion of pain relief or medical findings. There have been hundreds of books written about migraines. Millions of dollars have been spent on medical research. The result is a few helpful strategies for managing migraines, but to date, none of them amount to a cure for migraines.

My biggest concern with the current trends in migraine science is the focus on what is going on in your head. Once we realize that migraines are caused by an overload of toxins in the body, all this focus on the brain seems completely wrong-headed. I cannot fault the many brilliant scientists who have been trying to help. Since the major symptoms of migraine occur inside the head, it is only logical to start looking there.

The theory that toxins cause migraines is not new, but for some reason, it has not been a subject of scientific study. I hope this book inspires scientists to start testing this theory.

The relationship between migraines and toxins puts a new spin on the current approach to diagnosing and treating migraines. Here is a quick rundown of major trends from this perspective:

Pain Relief – Medications for pain relief are likely to damage your liver and should be avoided as much as possible. Natural remedies, such as essential oils and nutritional supplements, are preferred if they help.

Cardiovascular Medications for Migraine – Are also likely to stress your liver. Unless you need them for a heart condition they should be avoided.

Botox Injections for Migraine Relief – This is apparently effective for pain relief and probably harmless.

Migraine is a Neurological Disease – No. Neurological effects of migraine are symptoms of a systemic condition. The underlying condition is the body's inability to eliminate toxins.

If you are new to migraines or your symptoms have changed, you still need to see a neurologist. The symptoms of migraine can be easily confused with other serious medical conditions, such as a brain tumor.

Migraine is Genetic – There may be genetic tendencies toward deficiency in the liver and other organs that manage toxins. Genetic research has great potential for improving migraine treatment, but is still in its infancy.

I encourage you to do your own research and find out as much as you can about migraines. Keep track of your migraines and the remedies you try. Every migraineur is different, and the solution to your migraines may be the next big advance in migraine science.

Thank You

I am truly grateful that you took the time to read my book, and I hope you find this information useful. If I help even one person overcome their migraines then I have accomplished my goal.

If you have any questions, or if you want to share your experience with the cures I recommend, I would love to hear from you! Please email me at dawn@migrainecure.info. I usually respond to emails within one business day.

Before you go, here is a brief summary of my recommended cure for migraines:

1. Find a holistic practitioner to complement the treatment provided by your physician.
2. Take mineral supplements and drink more water.
3. Use Dandelion Root to restore your liver and clean your blood.
4. For intensive cleansing, try Yellow Dock on a limited basis.
5. Be good to your liver by eliminating bad fats, alcohol, sugar, and chemicals from your diet.
6. Use nutritional and herbal supplements to support all your waste-eliminating organs.
7. Take Dandelion whenever you are worried that you have triggered a migraine.

8. Drink more water. I can't say it enough. Water is the source of life and the source of health.

I am learning new information about migraines, toxins, and natural remedies every day. I am starting a newsletter and have several e-courses in the works. You can find out more by registering on my website http://www.migrainecure.info.

Finally, please take a few minutes to leave a review on Amazon so other migraineurs will know whether this book has been helpful for you.

Thank you and I wish you the best on your journey to becoming migraine-free!

Dawn Gregory
July 27, 2015

Index

27092324R00035

Printed in Great Britain
by Amazon